THE SINGLE MOST MPORTANT

Health Secret of All Time

Personal Testing Via Body-Energetics

The Breakthrough Way
To Make Optimal Decisions
For Your Health and Well-Being

Ronald M Bazar

The Single Most Important

Health Secret of All Time

Personal Testing Via Body-Energetics

The Breakthrough Way
To Make Optimal Decisions
For Your Health and Well-Being

Published by: Ronald M. Bazar, B. Com, MBA
Address: PO Box 73, Cortes Island, BC, V0P 1K0 Canada
Email: ronbazar@gmail.com
Copyright © 2017 by Ronald M. Bazar

Contents

Introduction

Recent advances in the new field of body-energetics (informed body energy awareness) make it possible for anyone to learn how to apply its principles in order to learn what is best to eat or do for optimal health and well-being.

Imagine having a simple tool or technique that helps you know whether a particular food or supplement is what your body needs.

It is important to remember that we are all unique beings with individual needs, and with that, our eating and wellness choices will be different for each of us.

The reality is that no one else truly knows what is best for any unique individual — at best, they can provide insightful guidelines for you to verify yourself or prove not useful.

We are complex beings and what works great for one of us, will not necessarily work for all of us.

This is where the diet and health pundits fall short. They are convinced that they have found the pot of gold at the end of the rainbow and they want everyone else to find it too. They may mean well, but to follow their exact method or product advice will not give everyone the hoped-for results, as we are individuals with unique needs.

You can understand now why this approach would not work for many people. We are just too unique, too complex and too individual for such a simplified approach.

What we need is a way to know for ourselves. We need an approach that allows us to know for sure.

Wouldn't it be great to know whether butter or margarine is

better for you?

Wouldn't it be helpful to have the knowledge to know if coffee is good or bad for you today?

You could easily verify if eggs are what your body needs now?

Or, is meat something you should eat or not?

Or, is this particular food causing you an allergic reaction?

Or, is this new supplement actually going to help you?

Or, is this practitioner someone who resonates with you?

What if there was a way to have the answers to these questions without a doubt?

Wouldn't that be invaluable to you?

The good news is that these questions and others you have about your health and diet can now be answered by you.

Advances in body-energetics allow you to personally test to know for sure, in seconds, the answers you need.

This will be a huge breakthrough for you and your health. You will be truly empowered and will have a tool or method to make your own optimal diet and wellness choices.

You will also save a lot of money not buying special foods or supplements that are not beneficial to you.

Have You Been Disappointed Countless Times by The Latest Weight Loss Book, Miracle Health Supplement or Diet Plan?

How many times have highly credible doctors and experts recommended their method as "THE WAY" to diet, wellness and weight loss success?

Have you spent a small fortune on highly recommended supplements and vitamins of all kinds, yet you haven't received the promised or hoped-for results?

Have you been tempted to try that new "miracle" supplement, claiming to have drastically changed the lives of so many smiling people…only to try it and be let down once again?

It sounded so good and so convincing that you went for it whole hog, but it didn't work.

Hey, I've been there and I've spent a fortune on promises that never worked for me. What about you?

Have you seen some of the latest ideas like the "**China Diet**" or the "**Paleo Diet**", or the "**High Protein No Carb**" Diets, or the latest trend, "**The Raw Food Diet**", or "**The Vegan Diet**"?

They each seem to make good sense with all the expert analysis, scientific facts and figures.

These experts tell you that all you have to do is follow their advice and you will succeed. The pounds will shed away "just like that", and you will enjoy "perfect health forever"…

You have been so let down. You've had your hopes dashed just like me. You bought in, tried it and it didn't work. You wasted so much of your time, money and energy.

It is not your fault. Sure, there may be some good ideas in these diets or health improvement books, and perhaps some excellent ingredients in the *"magic"* supplements that are highly promoted to cure what ails you.

BUT -

The reality is that *we are all so very different.* What works for you, may not work for me.

How can something work for all people, when we are each unique individuals?

The diet gurus and health pundits assume their plan will work for everyone else because it worked for them and their selected, successful patients.

We all have individual constitutions and conditions such that NO ONE diet, health supplement or health advice will work for everyone all the time, let alone be ideal.

So, what are you left with afterwards?

Disappointment, frustration and even anger at the lack of results never mind the loss of time and valuable money spent. What a waste!

You've spent a fortune and nothing has worked.

You see, it is not your fault if the choices you make are not the best ones for you.

You just don't have the proper tools to make the best decisions.

What you need is a way to KNOW what is best for you. Actually, truly, KNOW – at the core of your being, in advance.

So, is that possible?

If it were possible, it would be pretty useful, wouldn't it?

The new field of body-energetics makes it possible for anyone to learn how to apply its principles to the question of what is best for an individual to eat for optimum health and weight loss.

Sidebar:

I tried everything I could. You see, I was motivated…

I couldn't pee sometimes when I reacted badly to a food! I would have an extreme reaction that was life-threatening.

The wrong food could trigger my prostate to swell, blocking the exit of urine from my bladder and not a drop would come out.

So, began my quest for a solution without radical surgery, which would have resulted in impotence and incontinence and diaper wearing for the rest of my adult life. It is quite the story, believe me! (See my book *Healthy Prostate* http://healthyprostate.co/)

I was so motivated to succeed because having to use a catheter for relief was no fun, to say the least.

So I bought all kinds of health books, followed special diet plans from top natural health experts, ate the best organic foods, took the best natural supplements (as much as 24 2x per day), saw all kinds of alternative practitioners, the best homeopathic doctors, naturopaths, Traditional Chinese Medicine doctors, top natural healers, leading authors and practitioners of natural health and healing, bought more books and techniques and products, and on and on...in eight years I spent approximately $100,000!

I even tried attuning to my inner healers, guides and angels to help me. I meditated and I prayed.

I was desperate for a solution to my misery. I had no success, no matter what I did…

… until I discovered the breakthrough that I am going to describe to you here.

What if you had a way to figure out exactly whether something was good for you to eat? Wouldn't that be empowering and affirming for you?

I am not talking about making guesses here.

I am talking about really KNOWING.

That's a huge difference.

Knowing at the core of your being...

You could walk into your food store and be able to choose the foods that were ideal for you, right now.

Here's another thing. Everything changes. It's a law of the universe. Sometimes, positively and sometimes, negatively.

What is good for you this week or month could change and no longer serve you the same way it once did. And vice versa. Something that is not good for you today may be OK for you next month.

Sidebar:

I'll give you an example: cucumbers. I especially enjoy them in season, picked from my own garden.

But I was recently having both prostate reactions and stomach problems simultaneously, but I couldn't figure out what was causing it.

I finally decided to test every single thing I had eaten during the day, and low and behold, the culprit was cucumbers! I couldn't believe it. My own organic lovingly-grown babies did that to me?! So I cut them out, and now feel much better.

There is a way to <u>know</u> and there are simple techniques you can learn that tap directly into your inner body-wisdom.

We all have an internal guidance system. It comes with being human.

The problem is that we have lost the ability to tap directly into our **inner-knowing or inner energy awareness**.

We have become disconnected from ourselves and our inner-knowing, by way of the stresses of modern life, including a detachment from our roots with nature, information overload, technology and harmful environmental inputs.

We do not even know that there is now a method to access our inner body-wisdom quickly and easily.

These recent advances in the new field of body-energetics now make it possible for anyone to learn how to access their inner-knowing and make informed body-energy-awareness choices.

This is real empowerment that will change your life for the better and save you time, money and energy.

Just like it did for me, it will allow you to **be the master of your decisions**, knowing you are making the right choices.

You see, you and your body are a most sophisticated energy field. All you have to learn is how to properly tap into your inner knowing that is already there.

Anyone can learn this within a short time and you can watch your life shift for the better

This is not some wishy-washy *"new age"* or *"magical"* concept, far from it. My practical business background just doesn't allow me wishful thinking.

This is realizing that the human body has an innate wisdom that no machine or computer can come close to mimicking. The adage: "The Answer Lies Within" is so true.

With these techniques, you will KNOW and KNOW THAT YOU KNOW because you can tap directly into that inner knowing.

Now that is exciting, let me tell you!

It is easy to learn if you follow the simple instructions. One of the techniques even teaches you how to know if the testing you are going to do will be accurate and not give you a false positive.

So, with these simple techniques, you are the expert who KNOWS the answers directly.

Nobody else, just you.

That is so empowering!

I got so excited when I learned these techniques. I was able at long last to KNOW what would work for me and what wouldn't. At last I could discover what was causing my prostate attacks and the resulting pain and anguish.

For example, one simple thing was coffee.

How many conflicting reports have you read about the bean?

Some studies (https://goo.gl/chbUpo) say it is wonderful for you up to X number of cups a day and other pundits say it is the worst thing on the planet to drink!
(https://goo.gl/aAeeJM)

How are you to know when such eminent scientific doctors and health experts yield such opposite conclusions?

Well, I found out my answer and you will too.

(Some days it is fine for me to drink and others not, and decaf almost always – but that's me).

What about you?

And not just for coffee but for any food item, any health supplement or weight loss product. You will KNOW whether it is good for you or not.

You will be free of disappointment and regrets of valuable money, time and energy spent on things that don't work for you.

Each one of us is so unique that we need this method to KNOW what is best for us.

It will empower your life.

There is no end to how you can use the techniques to enhance your life.

The answers lie within and now you can tap into that **KNOWINGNESS** yourself.

Learn this simple technique and it will change your life.

The Body as an Energy Field

The reality is that there is a strong debate between those who claim we have an energy field and the western scientific conclusion that it does not exist.

This energetic self is accessed and explained in both Chinese medicine using techniques such as acupuncture, and by the Ayurvedic medical system of analysis and cure of the body-mind.

Proponents of both these age-old systems of healing utilise a form of holistic discernment and approach to their craft, and do not fit neatly into the western medical notions of materialism nor evidence-based outcomes in a way that meets empirical western medical standards.

Read more about it here:
http://energeticsinstitute.com.au/science-of-human-energy-fields/

Acupuncture is an example of using the body's energy field to effect change. Here's how it became introduced to America:

In July 1971, Henry A. Kissinger, Secretary of State in President Richard M. Nixon's administration, went to Communist China to prepare for a trip with President Nixon the following year as part of the efforts to re-establish relationships with that country.

"While in China, one of the accompanying journalists— James Reston of the N.Y. Times—had an acute appendicitis attack. Chinese physicians performed an emergency operation on Reston to remove his appendix.

After the emergency operation was completed, Reston was in extreme discomfort and pain. To give him relief, the Chinese doctors performed an ancient practice of inserting needles into special areas of the skin to safely deaden the pain. This is called acupuncture.

Although Kissinger was naturally concerned about Reston, he was also fascinated with this method of relieving pain by the use of inserting needles in a person."

Acupuncture consists of inserting small needles on the body at key energy meridians. It could be on the foot or toe to stop the pain in the appendix, as an example.

This approach does not jive with Western medical views of the body, but makes perfect sense if you understand the flow of energy in the body as do the Chinese acupuncturists.

We all have a sophisticated, powerful, built-in ability to know. Body-energetic testing serves to access our inner-knowing with the compatibility of the object being tested.

Historical Methods

In ancient and past times, sages and healers used dowsing with sticks and rods not just for water sourcing but also for placement of homes, temples, churches and sculptures.

You can study the precise use of sacred geometry in the exact location of many well-known places of worship, monuments, pyramids, art, and so on. My good friend writes about these in *Secrets in Plain Sight* *(http://www.secretsinplainsight.com/)*

We will explain much more in the next chapter so you can understand fully the world of Personal Testing and how it can benefit your life so much.

The Body-Energetic Secret Personal Testing

This material presents you with a tool that will enable you to know—with certainty—whether a food or supplement is beneficial for you to consume or not, right now. You will also be able to use the tool for many more areas in your life.

Your daily food is your most important medicine for optimal health.

It sure is wonderful to have a reliable way to **know** whether something is healthy for you to eat.

Look, this may not be for everyone…

The techniques to which I'm referring will be very challenging for some readers to accept, especially those of you with a scientific mindset. I know that personal testing could be easily dismissed as unscientific and not valid.

I believe this kind of thinking would be a mistake.

Why? Because I know it works and it has saved me, and many others, countless anguish.

I have had so many examples of being able to discover a problematic food or supplement, which — within hours of taking it — caused me very severe reactions, sometimes including the complete inability to urinate, as I have previously explained.

Testing that item before I ingested it would have been exactly the preventative measure that I needed to take to avoid the resulting pain.

I admit to being a slow learner sometimes, but if I have had a reaction, I have always been motivated and able to find the culprit that caused it by testing all that I ate in my last meal.

And many times I have stopped myself in advance from taking something that personally tested NO and thus was able to avoid those reactions.

Suspend your judgment for a moment if you want results.

Personal testing works, if done correctly. If you have a weight problem or a health condition, testing your inputs is a crucial step to stop the triggers that are worsening your condition.

Before I go on, let me tell you a bit more about myself.

I am a business graduate of McGill University and Harvard Business School many decades ago. I have a strong business and entrepreneurial background and I am often quite sceptical of the latest and best, as part of my critical nature.

So when I first was exposed to what I am about to share with you I was very sceptical, believe me! How could such a simple technique work? I was incredulous. Give me a break!

But anything that could prevent or save me from having to use a catheter in the middle of the night when I awoke and could not pee, forced me to suspend my scepticism and give it a try. I was starting to realize that something I ate could trigger an allergic-like reaction that caused my already enlarged prostate to react and make me unable to pee.

It was also life-threatening to me if I could not get the catheter all the way through.

Sometimes, with an extremely enlarged prostate, it squeezes the pee tube so tight that it is very hard to push the catheter all the way past the last critical bit through this swollen prostate into the bladder thus allowing an exit for the urine.

I live on a remote island and failure meant a long delay to get to the hospital and hours and hours of extra agony. This happened to me twice and I was screaming in pain from an about to burst bladder.

You could certainly say I was motivated to prevent that from happening!

So when I learned about personal testing I suspended my judgment and became curious.

At last, I had found a tool that worked to let me know if something I was about to eat would shut the door and leave me helpless and screaming!

(By the way, I have used all the insights from emergency room nurses and doctors, as well as tips I learned along the way to write my book: *Secrets of Male Catheter Insertion for Prostate Problems* (http://amzn.to/2c1Fyfk)

Sidebar:

Beep goes my email inbox of a new arrival from one of the foremost organic vitamin and supplement manufacturers in America…

I read headlines of the latest and best must-have antioxidants that will prevent disease and help you on the way to recovery of many health conditions.

Sounds so enticing because, heck, if it's true, why not? We all want better health.

Well, I will teach you how to know if that supplement is a buy or a pass-by for you.

I call it "personal testing" because you are testing whether something is beneficial for you or not.

It has other names as well: body-energetics, muscle testing, behavioral kinesiology, body tuning, energy testing, energy awareness, bio-energetic testing, bio-resonance, pendulum testing, personal dowsing and more.

Behavioral Kinesiology is an integrated system for assessing and evaluating the effects of all stimuli, internal and external, on the body, enabling us to arrive at a new understanding and synthesis of the integrative action of the body energy system.

http://www.icnr.com/articles/behavioral-kinesiology.html

If you have heard these terms before and have negative thoughts about them, please suspend your judgment and read on.

Yes, there are some people that use these techniques incorrectly, and that may prejudice your views. I understand.

But do hang on and realize there are proper and improper uses. <u>It is very important to learn correct methods.</u>

Read what Albert Einstein has said:

"I know very well that many scientists consider dowsing as they do astrology, as a type of ancient superstition.
According to my conviction, this is, however, unjustified....
Dowsing... shows the reaction of the human nervous system to certain factors that are unknown to us at this time."

Personal testing can quickly let you know:

- whether a food is good for you or not,
- whether a supplement is conducive to your health or not,
- whether a medication or herbal remedy is good for you or not,
- whether a body-care product is good for you or not,
- whether a household product is helpful to your health or not,
- how much of an item is optimum to take, and
- many more uses in your daily life.

Here's an example: I love chocolate! I have not been able to test positive for months and months. I go into the health food store and test their organic chocolates, and I always get a NO, no matter how much I wish for a YES! I gave up testing chocolate for about a month and, lo and behold, I am now getting a YES for 85% dark organic chocolate. YES!

There are many theories or facts about what you should or shouldn't eat. They can be excellent starting places for ideas and suggestions. But the final test is whether or not it is good for you.

All you need to do is be patient with yourself as you attempt to learn to personally test foods and products. It takes a little bit of time, but with persistence, you will develop a skill that is invaluable to have for your health. You will then **know,** what is good for you or not.

What is Personal Testing?

Personal testing involves tapping into your personal awareness or body-energy by using the techniques to access your informed-body-energy awareness, which then gives you the answer you are seeking.

We all have that internal guidance system. It comes with being human.

In an article entitled "The Intelligence of Your Cells," (https://goo.gl/A9mKU8) biologist Dr. Bruce Lipton, (http://www.brucelipton.com/) states that the conscious mind is capable of processing 40 nerve impulses per second.

But the subconscious mind can process 40,000,000 nerve impulses per second!

Hence, when you personally test, you tap into your inner knowing—your subconscious mind—and bring it to conscious awareness.

We all have this ability. The problem is that many of us have lost the ability to tap directly into our inner knowing. Modern life disconnects us from our roots with nature and puts stresses of all kinds on us.

How many times in your life have you said to yourself, "I'm full, I shouldn't eat any more," and then found yourself dishing up yet another plateful of food? You didn't listen to your inner knowing and ate more anyway.

We have trained ourselves to stop listening to our bodies' signals and needs. We ignore the feedback mechanisms that are meant to keep us healthy and in balance.

Personal testing gives you a way to tap into that inner

wisdom and to learn to listen to what is right for you in this moment.

This will help you to choose foods and products that are health-enhancing for you, to help prevent health problems and to help speed you on the path to recovery, optimal wellness and weight-loss.

Some readers may scoff at the techniques for personal testing, possibly because they think it is not scientific. What I can tell you is this: It has worked for me and for thousands of others — there is no cost or drawback to giving this a try.

With an open mind, try the techniques outlined here. Practice them in the quiet comfort of your home, with no one watching, and see what happens.

Sidebar:

Remember, we are electrical in nature. All our cells rely on an electrical charge to communicate with each other. This electrical life force is composed of positive and negative charges. The Taoist symbol of life shows this constant interplay between these polarities in the form of yin and yang.

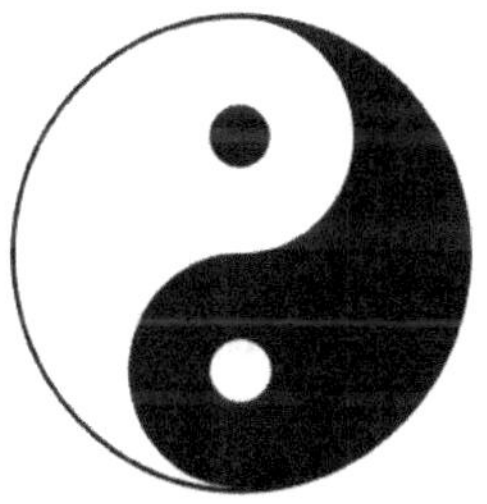

Perhaps it is the interplay between the electrical force of the thing being tested and our own cells that make personal testing work. Remember that in quantum physics the boundaries between time and space, matter and non-matter are non-existent, and so somehow we are able to connect and know if we tune inwards.

Perhaps a simple real world example can do. When we meet someone new, sometimes we find an inner knowing that that person does not resonate with us, or vice-versa. We are often simply picking up on unconscious vibes. But we know.

Look at what Dr. Joe Dispenza says in his amazing book, *Breaking the Habit of Being Yourself: How to Lose Your Mind and Create a New One* (http://amzn.to/2r2suP5)

We Are Connected to Everything in the Quantum Field

Like everything else in the universe, we are, in a sense, connected to a sea of information in a dimension beyond physical space and time. We don't need to be touching or even in close proximity to any physical elements in the quantum field to affect or be affected by them. The physical body is organized patterns of energy and information, which is unified with everything in the quantum field.

You, like all of us, broadcast a distinct energy pattern or signature. In fact, everything material is always emitting specific patterns of energy. And this energy carries information.

Thus, what you test emits its on vibe and interacts with your own energy to give you information about its helpfulness for you.

If these personal testing techniques work for you, then you

have gained an unparalleled tool that will facilitate your health and save you time and money. There is nothing to lose and everything to gain.

All I can say to you, dear reader, is that this skill has saved me from countless agonizing experiences.

I also saved a fortune not buying highly promoted supplements that tested NO for me. In fact, about 95% of promising, top-of-the-line supplements test NO for me.

If you are able to put aside your doubts and scepticism, and can give personal testing an honest try, I believe it will be a boon for you. It will take just a little bit of time and effort to get good, but it is so worth committing yourself to.

Luckily there are three basic ways to do personal testing, one of which will work well for you.

Sidebar:

When I get a NO for something that I like, I find it easy to let it pass. Somehow, the fact of knowing it is not good for me now makes it easier to forego. You too will find this attribute for yourself.

How to Personally Test

Three basic personal testing techniques that you can use to empower you are:

1. Muscle Testing with a Partner,

2. Personal Muscle Testing, and

3. Pendulum Testing

Eventually, as your awareness develops and your natural instincts and intuition are strengthened, you may simply know whether something is beneficial for you or not without using testing techniques. Your subconscious knowing has energized your body awareness and you are in touch with your answer within.

Personally, since I am a very visual person, I love seeing the results of a test and find pendulum testing to be my favorite method.

Others, who may be more attuned to sensations, may find personal muscle testing to be their choice, while others may enjoy and find they get the best response when testing with a partner.

Whichever test you end up attuning to, dedicate yourself to your practice. Tell your inner skeptic to take a sabbatical while you test-drive personal testing — the benefits are so worthwhile.

Personal testing has the potential to save you a lot of money because you won't buy products that aren't meant for you, at least at this time. You will be able to design your own perfect diet and choose only beneficial supplements, based on your own personal guidelines and inner-knowing, instead of relying on the expertise of an outsider.

I offer you these three methods so that you can find one that you like. Each method has slight variations. Just develop the skill with whichever works best for you.

Okay, let's begin!

{CAVEAT: These methods should not be used to exclude the proper advice of your healthcare practitioner or doctor.}

Muscle Testing with a Partner

Also known as *behavioral or applied kinesiology* or *muscle strength testing*, this test requires two people: you and your partner, who will test you.

Please note that this method is used by some health advocates or practitioners to test the health or strength of internal organs. But that, in my opinion, is an incorrect use of the method.

When used as I describe in my next section below it is a simple method to detect which food or supplement tests positive for you. That is all it does and should <u>not</u> be used as a diagnostic tool, as the well-known physician, Dr. Andrew Weil, (http://www.drweil.com/) says here, and I concur:

Dr. Weil notes that physiologically, there's no reason to believe that an external evaluation of a muscle's strength can diagnose nutritional problems inside the body, or that consuming a certain nutrient could immediately correct a severely weak muscle. He maintains that AK (applied kinesiology) falls far short on reliability for diagnosis and treatment of any health condition, and advises both skepticism and caution when it comes to this form of care.
Read more here: https://goo.gl/dLy4u8

Muscle Testing with a Partner

A quiet and calm environment is best.

1. Both of you stand. Let your left arm hang down comfortably at your side. Your dominant arm (for most people it is their right arm) extends outward in a horizontal position with your elbow fully extended. (If you are left-handed, reverse the arms.)

2. Have your partner stand behind you. Close your eyes, take a calm, slow deep inhale through your nose, into your belly, and out of your nose. Relax your mind. Your partner then places her left hand on your left shoulder to keep you stable, and the fingers of her right hand on top of your right arm over your wrist. Some prefer to face each other, but I think it is best to avoid visual contact.

3. Your partner will say, "Resist," and then press down quickly on your arm while you try to resist the pressure. Your partner should do this firmly and smoothly. It is not a contest but rather a way to notice if the arm remains strong or weakens.

4. Your arm muscle will test strong in this neutral state. If you are in an emotional state or under the influence of drugs or alcohol, it is not a good time to test as you could get mixed results.

5. Now we want to test something true. Your partner will ask, "Is your name [insert your name]?" Your arm should remain strong, which is a YES response.

6. Now your partner will ask a question that will give a negative response, such as, "Is your name Mary?" Your arm will become weak and will descend when pushed down on, which is a NO response.

Now you are ready to test a food or product. Hold the food item in your non-dominant hand (for most people this is the left hand) against your stomach area or solar plexus.

Then repeat the arm test. If the product is good for you, your arm will remain strong; if your arm is weak and it collapses, then the product is not good for you at this time. Now you have your answer.

In the case of a supplement that gave you a YES response, you then want to know how much to take. Here is what to do.

Start with one capsule in the palm of your hand and test again. If you get a YES, then try 2, then 3. Keep testing until you get a NO. The last YES is your dose for the day. You could take that amount spread over the day (e.g., take one supplement three times if you have three capsules as the daily dose).

In the case of a food like eggs that tested YES, retest with one egg then 2, and so on, to see how many you can eat.

It is wise to retest an item every day initially to ensure that it is still valid or that the dose doesn't change; this is especially important when you begin using new products or supplements.

For example, I started testing a new supplement that gave me a YES response.

The label advised 2 capsules per day, but I tested for 8! I obviously needed that supplement (cod liver oil)! That dosage lasted for a week. Through repeated testing, I started to reduce the dose per day down to 2 and then 1 capsule, and then, none.

You will have to practice the testing until it becomes easy

and natural to you. An open and calm mind is necessary when you do muscle testing. Remember your inner critic is AWL (Away with Leave)!

This Muscle Testing with a Partner Video is a good video to watch because it demos the basic technique. (https://goo.gl/qE1RNb)

Your arm muscles will respond to a particular item either with weakness or with strength, so long as you test properly.

Many foods and health products that seem irresistible based on their nutritious contents and marketing will test NO. I find that some wonderful sounding products do this sometimes *(eg. coconut milk)*.

If you test NO for a product that seems to have many "good" ingredients, it may be because one of the ingredients does not resonate for you.

Trust your test results.

Move on to something else. Your body may not be able to process or digest it properly, and you do not want to weaken your condition.

Later, when less sensitive, you may get a YES.

Please note that some naturopaths and other alternative medicine practitioners may use muscle testing on you to help them determine whether a particular supplement or vitamin or mineral is beneficial for you. This testing can be valid, but be wary if the end result is a huge list of products to buy from them. If you could learn one of the following methods, you could easily double-check those recommendations.

Personal Muscle Testing

If you don't have a partner to help you, you can still muscle test alone. There are two ways to do this:

Standing Method

Stand in a relaxed manner and repeat the word "YES" to yourself. Allow your body to move or swing you forward. Now repeat the word "NO," and you will find your whole body moving backwards.

Thus, by holding a food or supplement against your body, you will either tilt forward or backward, depending on your body's response to it. Does it resonate or not?

Try the name test: My name is [use your name]. You should swing forward a bit—YES. Then say something false: "My name is [use someone else's name]." The opposite now — NO.

You don't need to make the statements aloud—silently is fine. The idea is to train your mind for truth and falsehood, YES and NO.

Just practice this for a few minutes a day until it works for you.

Try some seemingly obvious items: see if Coca Cola gives you a YES or NO and then try an orange or carrot. You are ready to test now!

Here is a video for the Standing Personal Muscle Test. (https://goo.gl/ec87gP)

Finger Method

Hold the thumb and first finger of your left hand so they

make a circle (reverse if you are left handed). With the index finger of your right hand, you place it inside the circle and say YES, then pull it briskly outward (towards where your thumb and index finger are connected). You should test strong (YES), and you will not be able to open the circle. Now do it with NO and your finger should open the circle.

Do the same name test as above to get your YES and NO responses. Now you are ready to test.

You can then hold the product you want to test against your stomach or sternum using your arm while you then use your fingers to test. If it is a negative product, your finger will open and exit the circle.

Some testers use different fingers. Use what seems best for you. Here is a video for the Finger Personal Muscle Test. https://goo.gl/JCWqp7

Pendulum Testing

Pendulum testing is my favourite testing method, and I believe it can be the most accurate one if used correctly.

Pendulum testing requires the use of a pendulum to see your YES and NO responses.

What I particularly like is that there is a way to ensure you do not get a false test, like a false positive. That technique will ensure optimum accuracy of your results.

Pendulum testing amplifies your body's awareness and responses to what you are testing, and gives you a visual response.

While a pendulum can be made out of virtually any object that you can hang off of a string, better and more responsive pendulums can be purchased. I believe that getting the best pendulum is well worth the price of around $40 to $60.

The pendulum I bought was easily the best purchase of my life, saving me a lot of money on un-purchased, "great-sounding" supplements that tested negative, and even more importantly, saving me untold anguish of prostate attacks.

You could easily break-even the first time you go to buy a supplement that is supposedly great for you, and you test and get a NO, saving your purchase. You will then have recovered the price of the pendulum, and it's free sailing from then on.

Believe me when I say that most supplements will test NO not YES for you.

To avoid false positives and personal reactions to the device itself, select a pendulum that mimics the shape of the body's energy field, which is egg-like.

The reason is that this shape is optimum for testing. This eliminates many pendulums offered for sale in shops and Internet sites (pointy ones, strange shaped ones, long ones, etc.).

Here are some examples of pendulums I do <u>NOT</u> recommend:

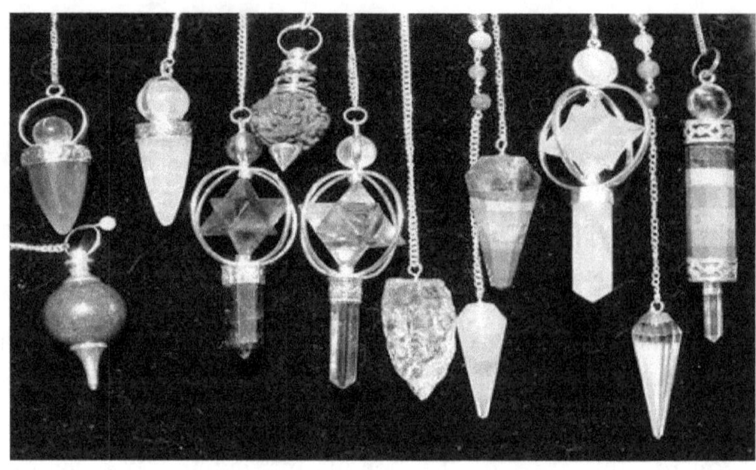

The most responsive and accurate pendulum-testing device is called the Omega Pendulum. (https://goo.gl/TqLpBF) The people who make and sell Omega Pendulums are experts in the field of personal energy testing with decades of experience, developing the finest testing tool you can find. I highly recommend these pendulums as they are the very best, period.

Watch this video (https://goo.gl/zntdjU) explaining the risks of improper-shaped pendulums for testing purposes.

Important:

In addition, your Omega Pendulum will come with a crucial piece of information — how to use the pendulum properly for accurate testing. This is most important as many people use pendulums incorrectly while asking it questions. This is not the way to test something. Please ensure you test correctly and do its self-test (from the instructions) to ensure no false positives.

Once you master using the pendulum, you can then graduate to using your body or hands as the testing device, even more accurately than the above methods. I still have a personal liking for seeing the responses, so I use my Omega Pendulum every time I test.

Even though some people can use a stone or exotic drop-shape pendulums like in that picture above, they can have a drawback of less accuracy by picking up environmental stresses that are weakening to you, and thus may give you a poor answer.

I have used many types of pendulums but none come close to the accuracy and ease of getting a proper response with an Omega Pendulum. (https://goo.gl/TqLpBF)

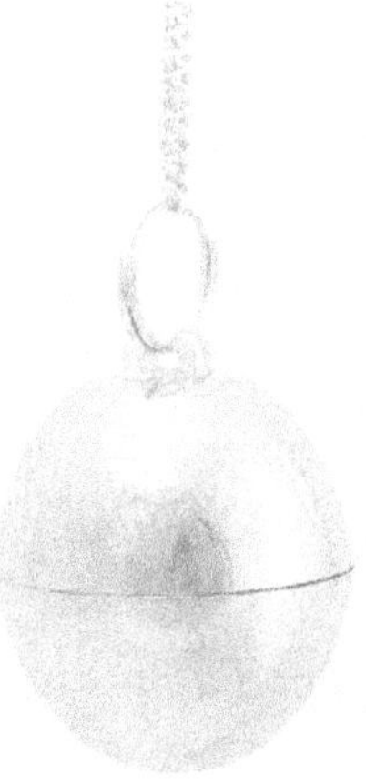

One of 3 colors of Omega Pendulums: Gold, Silver, Copper (https://goo.gl/TqLpBF)

The detailed instructions that come with it are equally as valuable as the pendulum itself. These instructions describe how to use the Omega for different kinds of testing that I have never seen done accurately with the other testing methods.

Keep in mind that you cannot ask a question when testing with a pendulum (a very common and incorrect use of a testing device). The proper technique requires getting a

direct YES or NO response to a product or image of it —
such as a photo — no questions asked.

Here is what the makers of the Omega Pendulums
(https://goo.gl/TqLpBF) say about it:

*The Omega Pendulum is simply an amplifier of your energy
body's response to whatever you are considering. The same
response is occurring even if you aren't holding a pendulum.
Never test with a thought in your head. Don't 'ask your
pendulum a question.' This will automatically bias the
response coming from your awareness and energy body.
Always keep your mind empty and let your energy body show
you what you need to do.*

*Instead of thinking, simply concentrate your attention on the
subject in front of you. Whenever you don't get a clear
response, let go of attachments to any particular answer you
might have and concentrate your empty-minded attention
more.*
Stephen Kane, Omega Pendulums (https://goo.gl/TqLpBF)

Below, I share with you a recent video I made in which I
demonstrate personal testing and how I personally test foods
and supplements with an Omega Pendulum.

Before you watch the video, I want to caution you that the
motions of your pendulum may be subtle at the beginning.
The turning may not be as strong for you as you see in these
videos (I have been doing pendulum testing for many years).
It may take time for your responses to become as powerful as
mine, but even a small movement YES or NO is

The Omega Pendulum is an improved and better pendulum
than the older version of the Perfect Pendulum also sold on
the website. The Omega is much easier to use.

Omega Pendulum Testing Video

(https://youtu.be/pykIV1ZJpH4)

Occasionally, you will get a neutral response, neither a YES nor a NO. Nothing happens or what happens is unclear.

With an Omega Pendulum (https://goo.gl/TqLpBF), a neutral response always means 'No' — the energy body is conflicting between a positive response and a reaction. But the inflammatory reaction will be triggered if the substance is consumed.

I recommend not eating or using that product unless you feel there is a good reason. When you are stronger, it will not matter as much. Retest that item later if you want to use it.

If you find you are having difficulties learning to personally test products, go to Food Energy Awareness Solutions and Training (http://www.feast.realhealth-online.com/) for an online consultation with the experts. They can help you learn with specific tips or by testing the foods and supplements that you want. Stephen and Lynda Kane are exceptional in this area. They are the ones who taught me and are the makers of the pendulum that I use.

Personal testing will revolutionize and empower your life.

Try to Set Aside Your Skepticism

I know, you're thinking that it's a bit too wacky for you and over the edge! This writer is too much!

But our subconscious knows what's best for us. Testing just tunes you into a conscious awareness of what you already know.

I know it is surprising, but this approach has consistently

worked for me. Many times I've tested an unopened product in a health food store that gave me a YES, and then retested the same product at home with the actual capsule in my hand, and I got the same YES response.

Personal testing has also worked on something that I sure wished was a YES, but I got a NO response. It was a super sounding prostate supplement, and I wanted to try it, but NO means NO, so I passed on it.

At times, I have taken a supplement that I didn't — or forgot to — test, because it sounded so good! But later it caused a reaction.

My typical reactions are either a sore tongue or frequent urination or worse—no urination, usually within hours, which indicates a severe reaction. Then later, after the reaction response, I test the supplement and get a NO. If only I had tested sooner!

If you have concerns about a personal bias, then consider muscle testing with a partner (as shown earlier in this chapter).

If you have concerns about people seeing you attempt this in a store, try the **Finger Method**, as this method can be very subtle. It looks like you're fidgeting, and no one will even notice you doing it.

Frankly, I don't care. I use my pendulum wherever. Most people do not even see you — they are too concerned with their own shopping.

I know it is hard to put your skepticism aside, but you have nothing to lose and a lot to gain.

Try it and see for yourself.

This has worked like a charm for me and saved me countless dollars and severe reactions, and I know it will work for you too.

Your body's inner wisdom knows what it needs. What you need constantly changes as seasons change, as you change, as your body heals and grows, as certain foods no longer serve you and new foods are needed.

So who are you to believe?

The latest scientific finding or study or some well-meaning health pundit, OR your body's own inner wisdom?

I know my answer and so will you when you learn how to tune in to your inner body wisdom. Use the good advice of others as a starting point to test against your own body's needs, and you will know.

How Do I Know Personal Testing Works?

Because I "back-tested" it. I believe my extreme sensitivities to many foods developed because my gut flora had weakened from

- vaccines, which weakened my body from the mercury and aluminum they contain
- antibiotics, which destroy good gut flora, and weaken immunity
- the removal of my tonsils when I was 8 which I now know from Chinese Traditional Medicine can lead to health problems later in life
- toxic heavy metals found in foods, supplements, water
- my many mercury fillings, which leaked minute

amounts of highly toxic mercury into my body over decades; and

- the anti-nutrient, phytic acid, found in many whole natural foods like grains, seeds and beans, unless reduced through proper food preparation.

I used to wake up in the middle of the night unable to pee— totally blocked! I eventually learned something had triggered the shutdown.

The way that I back-tested was by personal testing everything I had eaten at suppertime. I always found something that tested NO — the culprit!

So I started to test foods before I ate them. That was a simple, but effective, brainwave!

I had to give up all that I had learned about diet and the supposedly healthy foods with great profiles and scientific research that I was eating. The only thing that mattered to me was whether I would react to it — or not.

Real foods like my own garden kale, freshly picked apples from my own trees — and many more simple foods like organic brown rice — could block me tight so I had to use a catheter to pee.

I had just assumed that these whole natural foods could never be a problem! The same for the highest quality supplements. How could any of these be a problem? I was sure wrong!

Because my symptoms were so observable and so immediate, I became a living laboratory. My health was revolutionized by being able to personally test foods and supplements even of the highest quality and by discovering that many of them would not work for me.

By stopping all the irritants, I was finally able to stop the downslide and begin to heal. Now I can eat many of those former trigger foods.

Without personal testing, my condition probably would have worsened, and I would not have been able to find a way to stabilize and improve.

It can work for you too.

In my opinion, personal testing is the most important health discovery of all time, because it allows you to know what works for you — no theories, no guesswork, no must-do's.

You know. Period.

Personal Testing Theory

If you want to learn more about personal testing, read more in these informative books: *Your Body Doesn't Lie* (http://amzn.to/2hjjRbJ) ,
Energy Medicine (http://amzn.to/2cc5SRh) or
Muscle Testing (http://amzn.to/2bWxpL3).

And this book, *blinded by Science*, (http://amzn.to/2cEJstm) explains many mysteries of nature so you can understand how it works as well.

How personal testing manifests through a closed package or bottle, or even a photo of it, is a mystery to me but easily explained by quantum theory. I can live with uncertainty about how it happens because it has proven, without a shadow of a doubt, to work for me. It removes all the guesswork from my choices about other experts' recommendations. I just personally test each item and get my answer.

Testing Tips

If you are trying to assess if you can eat a certain food, don't ask yourself the mental question 'is this good for me?' Instead, just focus on the food and let your body energy awareness respond. Your Omega Pendulum will amplify this subtle energy response, giving you a clear Yes or No - no thought or mental self-talk involved or needed.
Stephen Kane, Omega Pendulums (https://goo.gl/TqLpBF)

When you get a YES for something new, retest it again regularly to ensure that the product is still good for you, especially if you have many sensitivities or if you are healing.

When I get a NO for a food, especially one that I like, I am happy to live with the decision because I know it is best for me. So I let any disappointment slip away quickly because I understand that I am benefiting by honoring the message in my body wisdom. My health will improve, and sometimes later on — I may be able to eat it.

You can do this too.

You can calm your mind and enhance your testing by placing the tip of your tongue up to touch the roof of your mouth behind your top teeth (an advanced meditation technique) and then swallow. Then test with whatever method you choose. When you get good at testing, it will only take a few seconds to get a response.

Instead of thinking, simply concentrate your attention on the subject in front of you. Whenever you don't get a clear response, let go of attachments to any particular answer you might have and concentrate your empty-minded attention more.

Remember no matter how "good" for you a food or supplement is, if you have too much of it, then it can easily change to "bad" for you! It has happened to me many times — with miso, sauerkraut, saw palmetto, selenium, greens, flax oil, my own tomatoes and more.

As you cleanse, detox and start to heal, your sensitivity to foods and supplements may go up temporarily. Your body knows what it needs. Set aside your opinions and personally test (and retest often). You will then know what is healthy for you to eat or not. As you get healthier and your sensitivity diminishes, you find that you have fewer reactions.

Using your energy awareness more, rather than just relying on your mind, feelings or intuition, will enable you to make many more energy-ascending choices in your life.

Trust your personal testing and avoid the reactions that a wrong choice can make.

Any food that you eat that triggers a reaction or that makes you feel unwell is something that you let slip through your defenses. Find and eliminate the culprit. Stop eating the suspect for 4–5 days. If you feel better, take that as a sign. If you then eat it and feel worse, then definitely stop.

But personally testing will save you the anguish. I always trust the test for it has proven to be 100% accurate for me.

When I forget to test and eat something that triggers a yucky feeling, I am always able to find it after by testing what I had eaten and forgot to test. Sure enough, the scoundrel is there.

I then avoid it and after quite some time will gingerly test to see if it's OK to eat some. Some foods may take months to eat again — or never — if they are a true allergen.

Remember we all have multiple sensitivities, not just to one food but several. Search and destroy, that is your mission!

Here is a tip. Test any new food that you think you want to try. If you get a Yes, eat it early in the day. Being sick at night is no fun if it triggers a reaction.

And here's another tip: sometimes you may get a YES for a new food item or one that tested NO before but now is YES. Be careful as it may mean a small serving size is OK or not very frequently. Start slowly. I have gone overboard when I finally got a YES to something that was a NO before. Don't be like me! I have too many faults!

Do not assume any food, no matter how natural its state, is safe for you to eat. Test <u>everything</u> as you start out, including your water and body care items.

I had always assumed that my own garden kale was a perfect highly nutritious food. It took me a long time of feeling worse and worse to finally suspect it. By then I was in a terrible state. When I tested what I ate at one supper, the kale gave a NO. At first I could not believe it! My own wonderful, organic, just-picked, super-green supposed super-food kale — could it be the culprit?! It was!

From the Omega Pendulum teachers…

Why Doesn't Everyone Know This?

Being aware of your own energy isn't 'scientific' because there is no scientifically-accepted definition of human 'energy.' Or any scientifically-accepted means of measuring it. Meanwhile, it just keeps doing whatever it happens to be doing - e.g. giving you a pain in the . . . because you just ate a food you are certain is 'good' for you - if you even bother to think about that question.

Unfortunately, even though almost all people are hypersensitive to some foods - which cause covert inflammatory reactions that eventually manifest as their symptoms or health problems - they usually have no idea which foods are harming them or which would help or heal them.

In fact, if most people really knew how their diet was affecting them - and acted accordingly - sales of drugs for arthritis, headaches, pain, digestive or neural diseases, psychological disorders, circulatory problems, skin conditions, behavioural problems, chronic fatigue - even cancer - would drop through the floor.

It's the proverbial 'elephant in the room.' Something that is massively affecting your health and well-being and is entirely under your control, remains almost a complete mystery - a mystery that can't be solved by reading about the latest 'superfood' or supplement, getting a PhD in clinical nutrition, paying a 'health coach' to tell you which supplements you 'should' be taking. Or, clearly, ordering an allergy IgG test.

Almost everyone ends up with physical or psychological symptoms or diseases resulting from repeatedly making food choices that cause sub-clinical inflammation. Energetic changes precede all eventual health problems, often by many years. It's prudent to nip problems in the bud. And these can only be identified by you becoming more aware of your energy.

But the fact is, contrary to popular, medical, 'scientific' thought, almost everyone reacts to some of the foods they eat on a daily basis; everyone's health is mildly or severely affected by what they eat; and everyone would feel considerably better if they really knew which foods work best for them. And which don't.

Since most cases of food allergy aren't diagnosed, the above assertion reflects the fact that there is no reliable scientific way to diagnose food allergies unless they are very severe, in which case an IgE test may be helpful. But for identifying more subtle inflammatory reactions to foods or other substances - which can still ruin a person's physical or psychological health or well-being through persistent symptoms or the eventual emergence of disease — nothing compares with whole energy body awareness.

Because it can't adequately be detected by scientific means, local hypersensitivity in the body, (as opposed to anaphylactic shock), is largely a 'non-subject' in medicine. This is based on the tautology that if an instrument can't (yet) reliably detect a phenomenon the phenomenon [therefore] doesn't exist. Or is of negligible consequence. This is equivalent to believing that before the Geiger counter was invented, radiation didn't make people ill . . .

The tragedy, from the point of view of preventing or recovering from illness, is that if medical science wasn't almost wholly instrument-dependent, millions of people would, at least, have the opportunity to recover from chronic symptoms or disease.

Stephen Kane, Omega Pendulums (https://goo.gl/TqLpBF)

Here are a few more uses of Omega Pendulum testing that come with the instructions for the pendulum:

- Is This Good for Me?
- Is This a Positive Remedy or Supplement?
- Is There an Environmental Stress Here?
- Life-Supporting Energy-Flow?

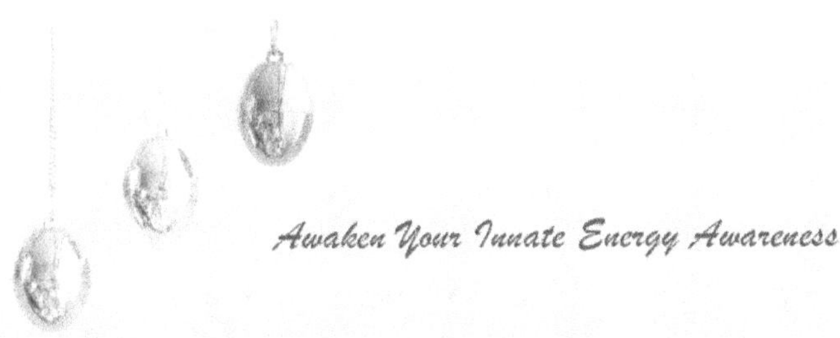

https://goo.gl/TqLpBF

I have used the pendulum for testing most objects in my home, new clothes whether to buy or not, a new book to read, a course to take, a practitioner to engage, cookware to buy or not, and many more daily uses. May you too enjoy the huge benefits of personal testing!

Now let me share some valuable insights from one of the originators of the Omega Pendulum as you step out into the new world of using your body as an energy awareness tool to help in your daily decisions:

Our mind is full of attachments, beliefs, information we gleaned which isn't true for us or accurate – what we call, 'illusory knowledge,' stresses, and other desires and resistances.

When you enquire of your energy body's wisdom (what you are doing when you use a pendulum), your awareness has to fight through all that lot of potential distortions too :) to be heard clearly by your mind as a YES or a NO. To pretend that we are a 'clean machine' when it comes to energy testing, capable of 100% detached neutrality about every decision we face is of course to deny palpable reality. Many dowsers never question the 'accuracy' of their dowsing, and thus don't develop their awareness very much – the whole point of using a pendulum. It's an awareness development instrument. A teacher if you will.

Imagine you know corn is no good for you. You're in a cafe with your older sister, you're starving, you do need to eat something, there's a delicious looking corn bread sandwich full of good things. Your sibling says she's going to have that. You can see a salad too on offer, you were considering that, but growing up, you tended to always do what your older sibling did – a lifetime habit, well embedded, perhaps unconsciously, in your energy body. And there was also a 'cultural value' in your family about fitting in and not making a fuss about your self. . . also still deeply embedded in your energy body/field, perhaps unbeknownst to you.

So . . . you test and lo and behold, it seems OK! So you eat it and then a few hours later feel rubbish and have stomach pains. Or, you don't bother to test, you just tell yourself, 'oh once won't matter, I've been really good avoiding that.' Or, 'oh, I'll just have what she's having' – obeying the two above somewhat unconscious imperatives. Same result though, whichever way you avoid your own awareness.

Then you can:

Beat up on yourself for 'getting your test wrong'.

Tell yourself this energy-testing game is obviously very unreliable.

Tell yourself I'm clearly useless at using a pendulum, may as well forget it.

Start double and triple checking all your testing (the mind loves to make people do this one).

or

You can say, 'Hmmh, that was interesting, I guess my awareness was overridden that time by some attachment or resistance of mine.' I'll really try next time to be as detached and still as I can be when I'm testing - in the presence of my sister particularly.

And maybe you even become aware of what the stress was... 'Gosh, I did it again, I just followed my sister's lead instead of doing what I needed to do. I'm going to keep an eye on that tendency'. (This is one-way awareness can be cultivated).

So, what about that tendency to want to double or triple check your test - it's best just to test once, then go with the result – or decide to ignore it :) At least that's clear and honest. :) some people's reason for retesting is that they don't trust themselves or because they want to get a certain result. Repeated testing of the same thing gains nothing. Your energy body has already responded to the best of its ability. Repeatedly doing the same test just degrades its usefulness. It's almost like your energy body is saying, 'Duh? I just gave you an answer to this?? Why are we testing again?'

Continued use of, and practice with, a pendulum brings you into a different relationship with yourself, one where you begin to trust yourself and your decisions and awareness of what is right/wrong for you. That journey can involve some deep stripping away of 'stuff' and many scales dropping from one's eyes. The pendulum is simply a tool in this process of coming into alignment with 'who you really are' and knowing what you really need.

Living with energy awareness will present you with the

current limit of your comfort zone and invite you to go through that – which of course means challenging some of the things I mentioned above, to which we are often very attached.

The funny thing is… people (without pendulums or any inkling of energy awareness) make a zillion decisions each day and never stop for one moment to worry about whether they made a right or good decision. But as soon as they start trying to be a little more aware of their decision-making, impossible standards of perfection and accuracy raise their head! 'If I'm not 100% accurate – i.e. all my decisions turn out good for me – then I'm not doing it right.'

It's a step-by-step journey. If your decision-making becomes just 1% more a reflection of your real needs than it was yesterday, that's huge progress.

Have fun exploring your awareness and your blocks to your awareness with your pendulum :)

Lynda Kane, Co-founder of The School of Energy Awareness, (http://www.eat.energyawareness.org)/) teacher, practitioner and energy-aware life coach and personal/spiritual development mentor

Conclusion

Each one of us is so unique that we need a personal testing method to **know** what is best for us. It is easy to learn one or more of these methods. This new skill will empower you to make better health decisions.

Personal testing will revolutionize your health by allowing you to test the advice and recommendations of others to find what works for you.

Personal testing leaps beyond the selling points of a well-marketed product or the ideas someone else has for you about what you "need" or what you "should" eat. Testing allows you to know for sure.

Take all the good advice that comes your way —from highly qualified health practitioners — and put it to good use by testing and making decisions based on your true knowing.

The only thing that matters is whether it is compatible for you or not. We each have an inner wisdom that knows just what we need. For me, that negated many recommendations from those experts. I got a NO to many of their products.

By stopping the inputs that rob you of your health, you take the first step to connect with that inner knowing.

Welcome to the mastery of your day-to-day choices!

Here are some action steps:

- Try muscle testing with a partner as a start to learning personal testing. Remember the test is not a contest. It is just to show whether something weakens you or strengthens you. Add the tongue tip described earlier.

- Be persistent and consistent so that you get better with whichever method you choose. Tune inwards and you will know.

- Try testing a few food items that you suspect are good for you and see if it confirms that.

- Try testing a few suspicious items next.

- Practice testing your inputs daily and make personal testing a routine part of your life.

- Replace depleted and toxic unhealthy foods with quality ones that you test.

- Now you can customize your diet in real time as your health requirements evolve. You can always be eating optimally while at the same time adjusting for social and personal realities. Perfection is not the goal rather just a healthy diet that suits **you** more and more over the years to come.

Invest in an Omega Pendulum (https://goo.gl/TqLpBF) if you want what I consider the best personal testing method. It is guaranteed for a year so you have lots of time to check it out. I am convinced you will agree with me that it is the most important purchase I have ever made.

Eating the foods and taking only the supplements that are positive for you will set you on the path to a life of improved health and wellbeing.

You too will discover that personal testing is the single most important health secret of all time.

About the Author

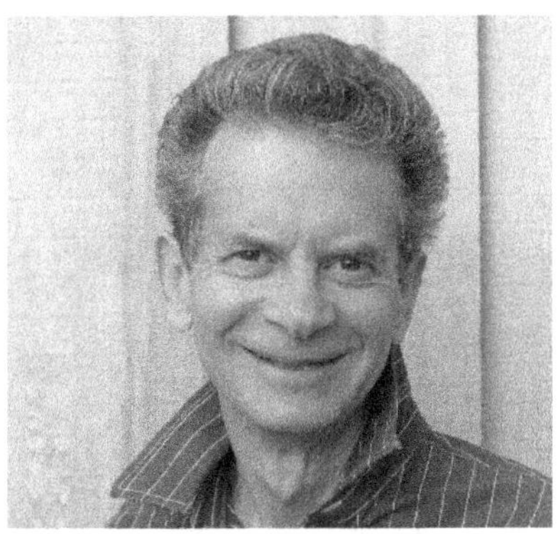

Ronald M. Bazar, a Harvard MBA, is a natural health enthusiast and author of seven books on the prostate including the comprehensive book on the prostate called *Healthy Prostate: The Extensive Guide to Prevent and Heal Prostate Problems Including Prostate Cancer, BPH Enlarged Prostate and Prostatitis*, (http://healthyprostate.co/) which is available on Amazon, iTunes, Kindle and more outlets.

He also authored *Your Perfect Diet: How to Customize Your Diet for Weight Loss and Great Health* (http://amzn.to/1JzOaXr)

and another well-received book:
Sleep Secrets: How to Fall Asleep Fast, Beat Fatigue and Insomnia and Get a Great Night's Sleep.
(http://sleepsecrets.co/)

Books by Ronald M. Bazar

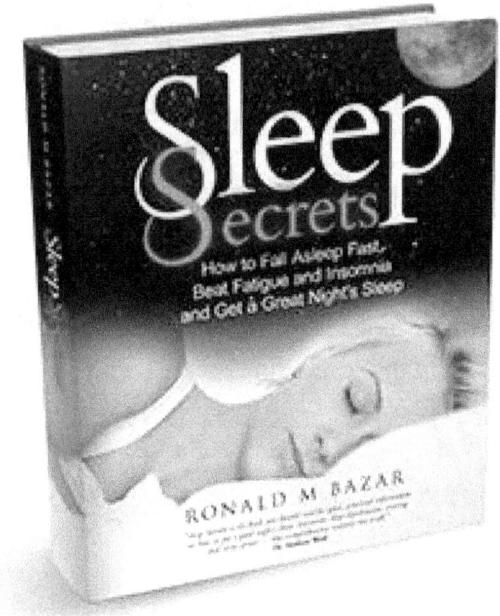

http://sleepsecrets.co/

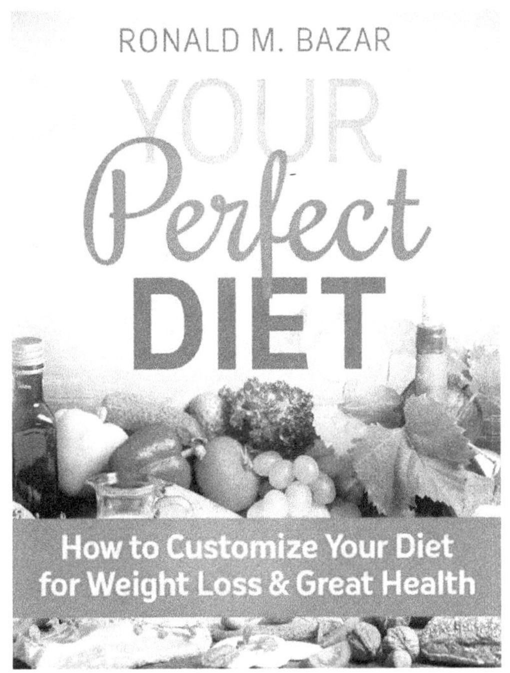

http://amzn.to/1JzOaXr

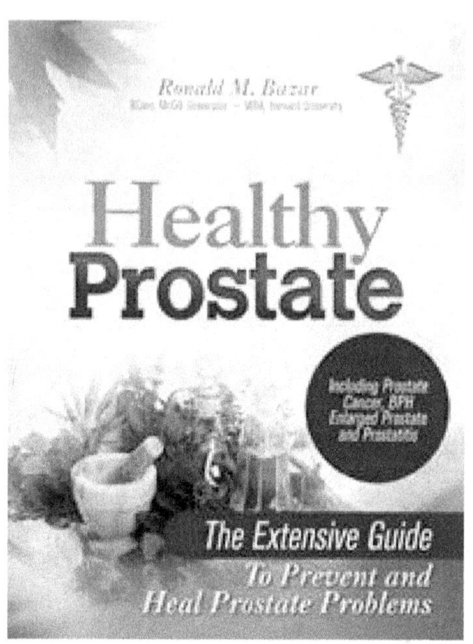

http://healthyprostate.co/

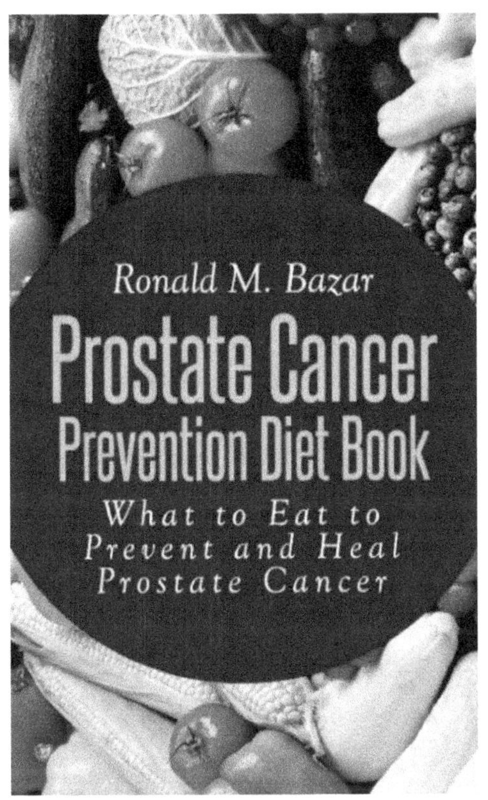

http://prostate-cancer-prevention-diet.com/

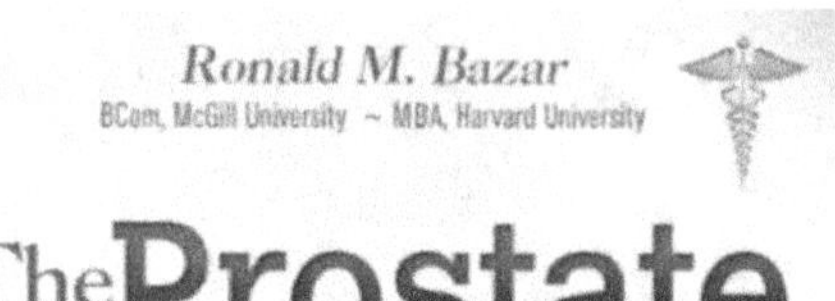

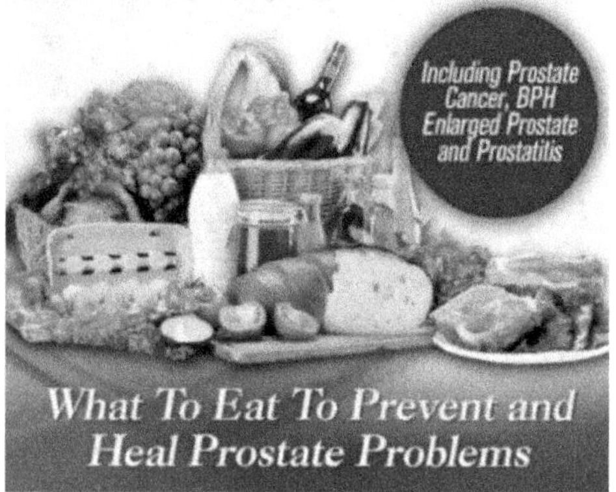

http://prostatehealthdiet.net/

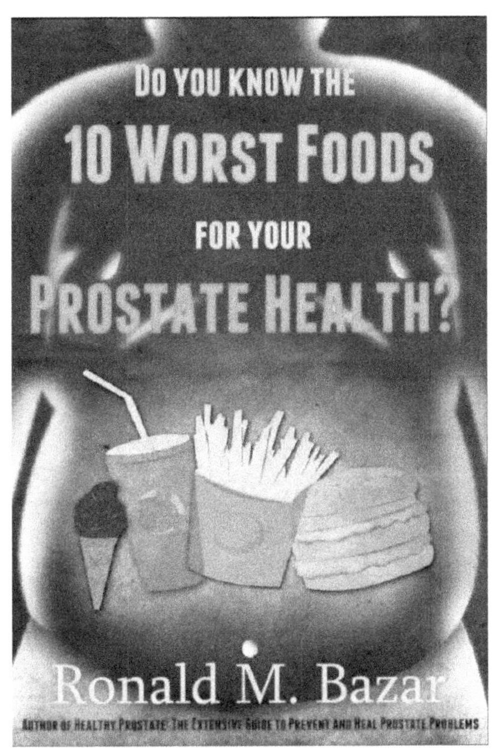

http://amzn.to/29hXPUY

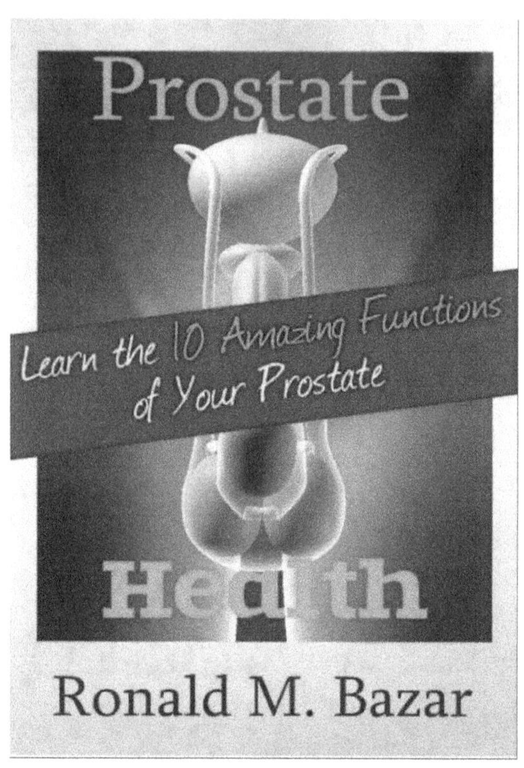

http://amzn.to/29hXyRV

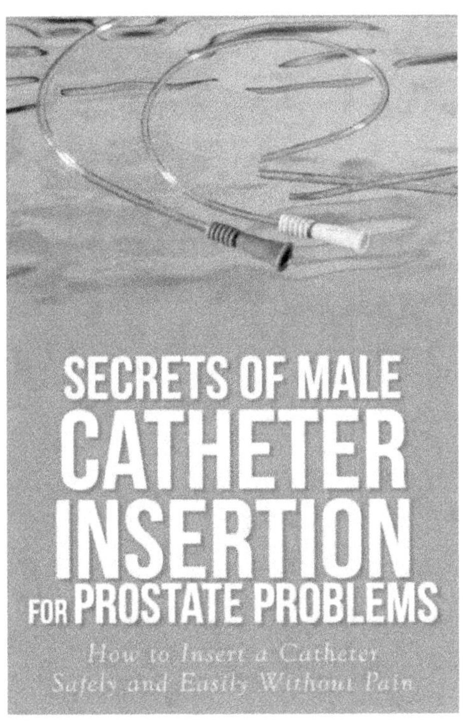

http://amzn.to/1S7uDkh

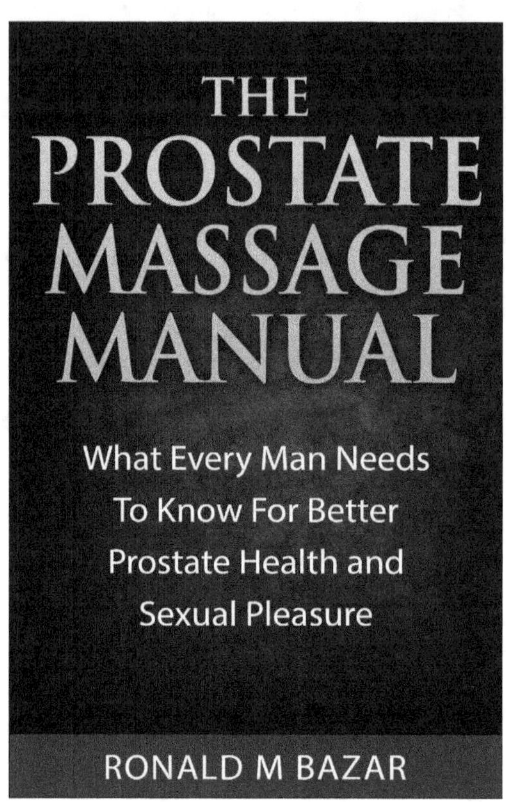

http://prostatemassagemanual.com/

Other Related Books

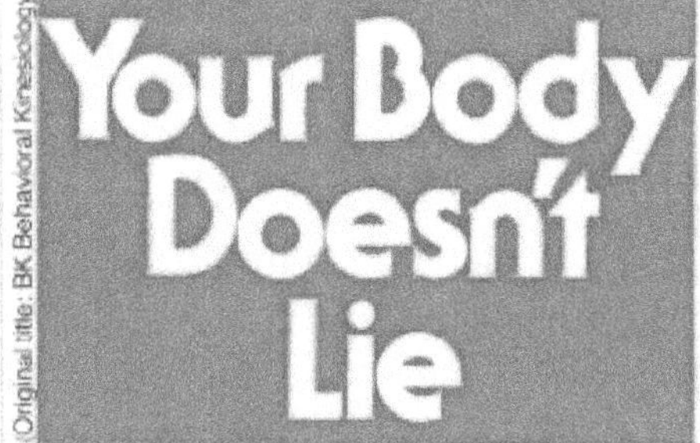

http://amzn.to/2hjjRbJ

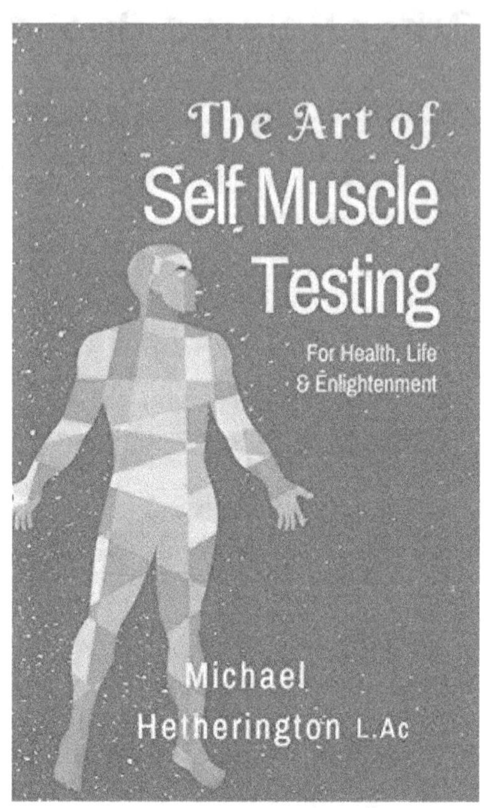

http://amzn.to/2g8Hztz

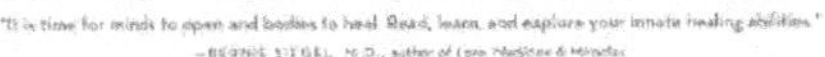

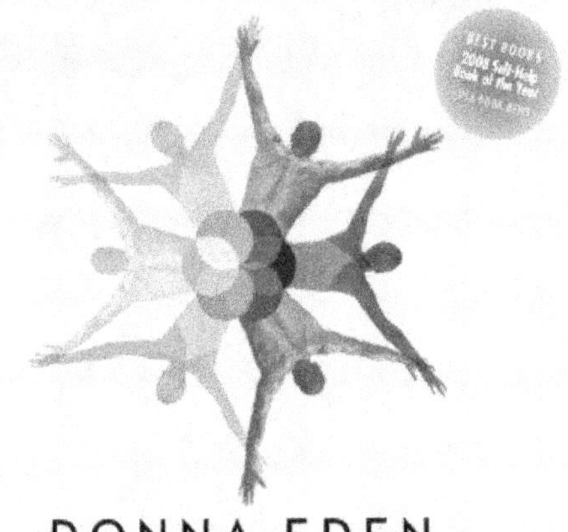

http://amzn.to/2g8Nui4

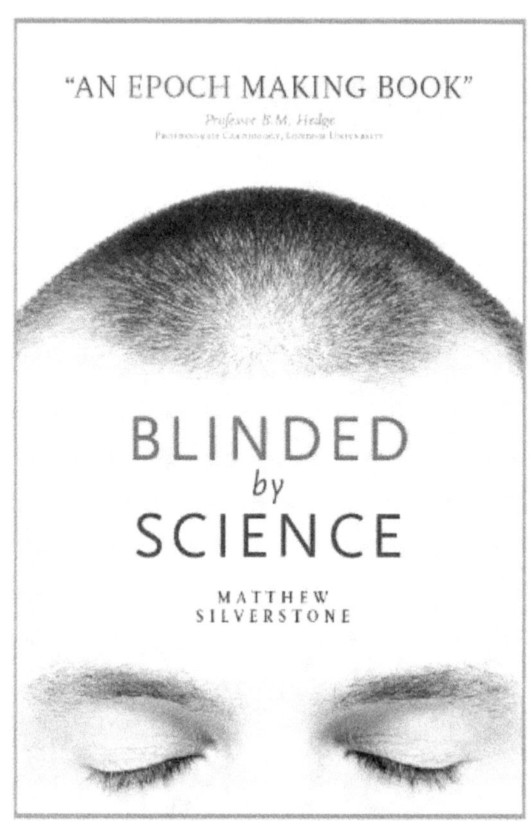

http://amzn.to/2gliLz1

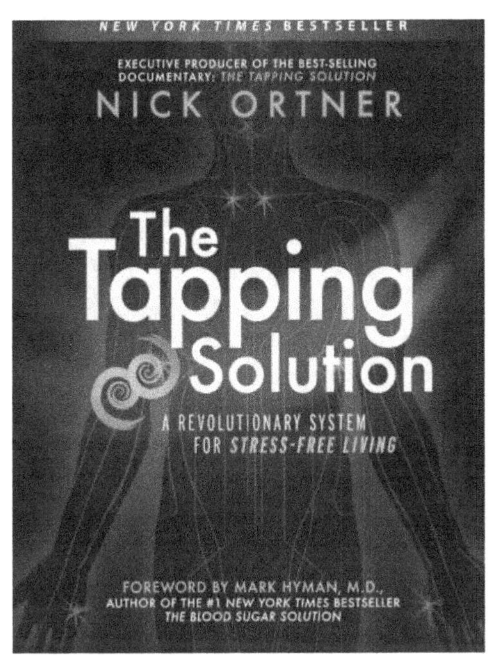

http://amzn.to/2hdDMeu

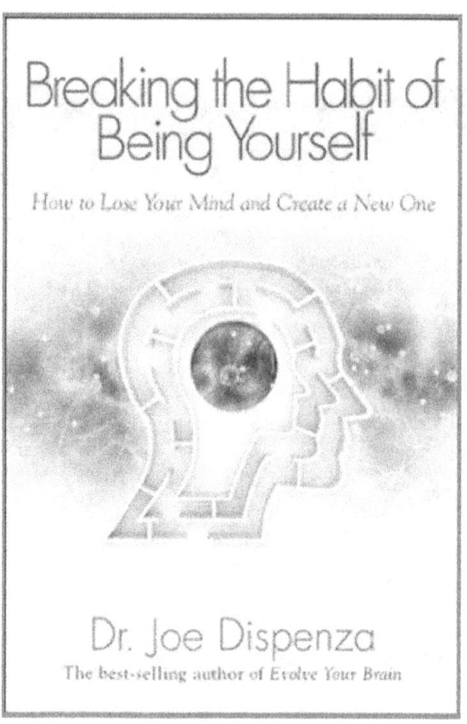

http://amzn.to/2r2suP5

Introduction

The world has changed so much since 2000 that we cannot imagine what it was like just a few short years ago.

Internet everywhere, supercomputers in our pockets now known as smartphones, instant communication, smart homes, internet of things, electronic and online games, e-movies, e-TV, videos all instant and now, smart devices, smart machines, wearables and apps for everything — your camera, video recorder, hand-held computer, and your lifeline to staying in touch with your work and family.

Life has changed, empowering us, enabling us, mobilizing us, instant everything, everywhere and always on.

We have devices now for sleeping, for waking, for cooking, for cleaning, for shopping, for playing, for delivery, for travelling and virtually all aspects of life with a waiting revolution still to come in the form of virtual reality, AI, and robotics that may be bigger than what has already happened.

We love our smartphones, tablets, apps and devices. They help us, entertain us and thrill us. We are connected and empowered.

The questions not being asked seriously enough are these:

- Have our standards of safe levels of exposures to the electromagnetic radiation they all emit been updated to protect us from a level of exposure millions of times higher than just a generation ago?

- What are the cumulative health consequences of this revolution in technology?

- What don't we know but assume is OK?

These are important questions because we just could be facing health issues that could overwhelm us in the coming years or decades.

Why?

Well, some people are already experiencing very serious health issues that can only be explained by exposure to electromagnetic radiation. They could be warning us like the proverbial canary in the coal mine of a disaster about to unfold.

There is just too much evidence proving the risks are very real for us to ignore. Yet it is not in the interests of the businesses that make the products nor in the governments that regulate us to pay heed to the hazards and in fact do the opposite by implying "Don't worry; be happy!"

There is no proof that Electromagnetic Radiation (EMR or Electromagnetic Field [EMF] Radiation) is harmless, certainly not in the doses most of us experience now daily. Long-term exposure health hazards are what we need to be concerned about because that is what we all risk by integrating our devices so thoroughly into our lives.

In fact, EMF radiation has been shown to affect living tissues and cells as well as our DNA in the brain and other parts of the body in direct close exposure to the radiation. Especially vulnerable are babies, children and teens.

The purpose of this report is to give you the information about the risks so you can decide if the evidence is significant enough to take seriously. If so, you will find many ideas on what changes you can make so you can still benefit from the convenience and enjoyment of your devices but can protect yourself from the possible health consequences.

Only you can decide whether to Smarten-Up and be a SmartBlocker!

Note dear reader:

if you want to get on the mailing list for this new book then go to SmartBlocker.co (http://smartblocker.co/) and sign up.